THE NANCY
REAGAN
COLLECTION

FUTUREPOEM BOOKS
NEW YORK CITY
2020

THE NANCY REAGAN COLLECTION

•

MAXE CRANDALL

first edition | first printing

This edition first published in paperback by Futurepoem Books
P.O. Box 7687 JAF Station, NY, NY 10116
www.futurepoem.com

Executive Editor: Dan Machlin
Managing Editor and Copyeditor: Carly Dashiell
Associate Editor: Ariel Yelen
Editorial Assistant: Aiden Garabed Farrell
Guest Editors: Pierre Joris, Claudia La Rocco, Monica McClure

Cover design: Everything Studio (everythingstudio.com)
Interior design: Nikkita Cohoon (ritualmorningstudio.com)
Typefaces: Futura PT, Mrs. Eaves, and IBM Plex Mono
Printed in the United States of America on acid-free paper

This project is supported in part by the New York State Council on the Arts with
the support of Governor Andrew Cuomo and the New York State Legislature. It
is also supported in part by public funds from the New York City Department
of Cultural Affairs in partnership with the City Council, as well as by The New
York Community Trust Harris Shapiro Fund, The Leaves of Grass Fund, and
Futurepoem's Individual Donors, Subscribers, and Readers. Futurepoem books
is the publishing program of Futurepoem, Inc., a New York state-based 501(c)3
non-profit organization dedicated to creating a greater public awareness and
appreciation of innovative literature.

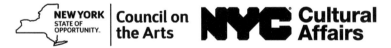

Distributed to the trade by Small Press Distribution, Berkeley, California
www.spdbooks.org

CONTENTS

•

1 | RED RIBBON

13 | FREE ASSOCIATION

23 | DAZED, FROM WHICH DISTRACTION

31 | ALL WAYS, A HUNTED

43 | JANET SPEAKS

51 | MY OWN PRIVATE PARADOX

59 | IRRESISTIBLE FORCES

75 | JUST SAY AIDS

89 | SWORN TO SECRECY

99 | AMERICA'S BRAIN

119 | MOTHERS AND LOVERS

127 | NANCY AT NOON

143 | FOOTSTEPS IN THE DARK

151 | MICHAEL JACKSON'S *THRILLER*

169 | NANCY AT BULGARI

175 | NOTES & SOURCES

RED RIBBON

•

Her gown's
a real sizzler

floor length
Bolshevik with
high-beaded collar

my little Galanos
nesting doll

Nancy Reagan
before me
in the
avant red
I adore

and shy away

What's a little haute couture to the woman who denies everything?

Trippy kitten telephone wires
lead me back to the bunker
choir, my secret rage

From here
I remind Nancy   on hold
allegiance comes with a price

Signed with a nice   *love always*

"I voted"

I can no longer give blood

Right into the future
what Nancy wears influences everything

Even me her groping styles determine all for instance
which window I open on which side of the house

What is for her
a simple choice—

pussy-bow blouse

in nautical theme

worn in a waltz across White House sod—

a yawn toward the
helicopter, her strident pilot,
uncertain hand shading his eyes

Contingencies like these   dictate my week's reading

Soul on Ice, Lolita,
a dash of Dickinson

Consequential events demand I take up tennis

possibly build a barn

Inside the barn, I discover
~~reading tea~~

~~verbena sacrifice~~

~~Mars in retrograde~~

~~shadow spells~~

4

Before long I learn to call her on capture

conjuring distant spirits

as if aircraft travel

gallant, as if

Through Nancy, I begin to see behind the image.

Not paranoia but the comfort of another dimension growing out behind this one starts to soothe pains, suggest lovers to me. So elemental, our one and only catalyst is allure.

Eventually my agenda becomes a shadow of what it once was

Dear North Americans,

I collect Nancy Reagans. Will accept doubles.
Payment in advance.

Seeking red ladies, vacation maidens,
stationary Nancys. Those who read written upon.

Will consider
damaged Nancys

even those involved
in her hasty
departure,
in May of '87,
to yellow.
Those aren't her, aren't really Nancys.

The wind is our streets, a romance behind us.

Love, Satan
(just kidding)

S A T A N

In 1991 AIDS takes on the color of her party: a right republican red. Everywhere I looked for AIDS I'd find Nancy Reagan, in any of her elegant gowns.

In one unblemished glossy, she reclines
across a plush red couch

our drowned mannequin
washed to shore

prostrate in pointy shoes

costume blazing

and braided
one over the other over the other

her stilted pose

sudden alarm on her face

her maddening inability to lounge

At the center of her coil
that murderous pillow lies

embroidered
like a gravestone

R period R period

The live self blinks behind the one represented

the self that knows its other

Nancys

My questions emerge

one

then

two

slimy
bubbles

flubbing
up against

the hopeless era

What self is saved?

What self wants to save?

I'm no Prince Charles but

I sweat

hallucinate

I swear on my life I once overheard

why this fierce attachment

Ronnie request

of Nancy's bewitching

fascination

Won't you, Mommy,
my little devil,

slip into something
a little more

red?

The banality of AIDS strips the epidemic of its political and personal emergency; it shifts the drama inherent in all experiences of AIDS, regardless of status, from the deadly serious to the almost trivial. AIDS is represented as trend, as fashion, as style.

—David Román

What happened was like an accident, a collision.

—Kimberlé W. Crenshaw

FREE ASSOCIATION

•

On the title track of her breakthrough album *Control* (1986),
Janet Jackson speaks: "This is a story about control.

My control. And I've got lots of it."
Everyone has a moment when they won't go back,

when *shh* becomes shove, double for nothing.
Mine is also a story about control,

about reading everything there was to know.

Most of what we could control early on
became known to us through speech,

small bites of knowledge shared aloud,
difficult to digest

without devising

otherworldly
ways of remembering

[Nancy Reagan with William Novak. *My Turn: The Memoirs of Nancy Reagan.*]

Her marriage: March 4, 1952. Her litany: *My life really began when I met Ronnie. I don't want to do anything else except be married.*

He and I both scoured the papers;
our textures enveloped neoteric language.

Dropping courage
down low

we jumped
the yellow curb.

We skipped and screamed through everything sealed.
What were we before or within, this uneasy arrangement?

Whereas ritual
mimics magma

a single me flows
tributary and Roman
toward the dancers

the moves
who follow
the madame

the mother me

and the witness
of the quick and flash—

the child emperor

A MOMENT   The two of us (me + my doppelganger,

twin flames)   sit alone in the Café Morocco,
          early afternoon.

     A quick brunch, leaning back in the booth, always
     helps us calm down, set right without that lasso

     in our throats: "In the old days, what did you think
     about the role of sentiment in film, especially for

     actresses searching for truth?"

Acting is what we had in common.
And the erroneous assumption that

the longue durée of our lives would consist,
primarily, of flouting the rules.

We'd seen *Lady Sings the Blues* (1972), our travel
built networks, all wise in the ways of Earth;

I had friends with friends on a leash.
This sacred center is where we lived now.

And him. My destiny, my one and only
glove clasped in the oval of my palm—

[Kitty Kelley. *Nancy Reagan: An Unauthorized Biography.*
Bedroom.]

Nancy's three months pregnant when they marry. Her mother Edith is an actress, a
figure straight off the stage of *Gypsy* (1962), who remarries before Nancy turns 10. Her
betrothed? Loyal Davis, a respected Chicago doctor with right wing tendencies. Nancy
and Ronald request a modest wedding present—a video camera.

To trace the uplift, so symmetry, of his face
when his lips parted. He was about to speak,

to say *me with you* at me, a song and an ask.
But shutter flash through the window

glaring with day, there she was. Nancy Reagan,
the high queen of Sacramento, rushing by on the street.

[1943 Smith College Yearbook, embossed.
Box Bin 1, wrapped in brown blanket.]

She is a size 4 her entire life. Neither Barbara Bush nor Betty Ford can stand her. For
at least eight years, Nancy's staffers try to broker an honorary degree from her alma
mater, Smith College (Class of '43). The more she wants it, the more it seems impossible
to secure. So Nancy skips her reunions, makes no donations, and ignores the tradition of
First Ladies extending White House invites to alumni. By the time Smith offers the honor in
1990, Nancy frostily declines.

Betty Ford studied dance under Martha Graham at Bennington. Pinch me, I'm warm.

Right there at the intersection of our three lives,
my muscles locked down and closed forever,

helpless and beating around
the one woman who could

ROCK HUDSON OCT 2 1985

In the flash I couldn't tell the difference.
Change became my life force, my magnetism

a dream, that dream became him, the annals, another me.
This excess belongs symbolically to Nancy.

My selves were a bundle I offered again and again.
In response, she introduced me to everyone, one flower
    at a time.

SYLVESTER DEC 16 1988

DAZED, FROM WHICH DISTRACTION

•

(Mouth of the Hudson)

Over the year Gipper rooted for me

—he really was—

considering how weak I'd become

something of a mirage

is being deserted

both miasma and

mise en abyme

his concern a canopy

I was held beneath

Violence is violence nonetheless

I was beginning to stoop low on account of my accident
near El Cielo

Thus encumbered I rode the Staten Island ferry nearly
every day to work

From my window I studied souls angling up   into arch

my mustache if I grew one

Back then I was entirely advertising and opera

disco and drugs

serenely composed

if little thought

in company

beside them danced

what I imagined was an escape

so many times before

There was what we called a mouth hole in the back room

I prided myself on hardly ever opening my eyes

One time I smelled gasoline

its sharp erasure

It was just like me

to be a midtown janitor

beaten to a pulp

after work in the dark

Nowhere to go again and

BOOM

that's when the market crashed

Suddenly the bars were empty

When I met him

I was limping through

—a bandaged risk—

talking to anyone who could listen

with people who didn't exist

The way she looked in me and smiled

the Gaze

Here was the Brutus apocalypse to keep us grounded

cord connecting face to air
Thoughts were coming like a pump where the rhythm made more
sense than the how

the high why

We possessed no ideal

no vision of what

overtopping loss

across the banks

would look like

Within that horizon

the people you loved became the people you hated

what you hated slipped in where you loved

Isn't it funny—it's always been that way for me:
At very emotional moments in my life it's as if I'm in a daze.

I fell for him as quickly as the sickness

Whenever he made a move

he had a custom of pushing his long slope of cheek

toward the nearest exit

Then, one day

the surgeons informed me

with great enthusiasm

We're rigging him up a brand new stomach

ALL WAYS, A HUNTED

•

In between the Nixon gigs that took them around
the globe for free, Nancy needed to get things done.

Right and left, putting the help in a hand
basket and playing a show to the owed.

CHARLES LUDLAM MAY 28 1987

Since meeting Nancy I'd had the distinct pleasure
of landing on the shores of Hell, so to speak,

where demon people profit from doom.
This was a dense area to cover on foot,

peering out of the eyes of someone
who was supposed to be me.

It was urgent to see what I could find
in a maze covering names in a feeling of politics,

to ascertain my weaponry within
this series of berserk emergencies.

[Photo w/ caption "Fixed bayonets for Bayview-Hunters Point occupation." Newsprint.
File Folder A-4.]

Ronald Reagan wins the California governorship thanks to white backlash in the state.
On September 27, 1966 (Watts Rebellion August 11-16 1965), a white police officer
murders Matthew Johnson, an African-American teenager, instigating the Hunters Point
Uprising in San Francisco.

Research: what is the toll of indirect witnessing? Where does this story belong? Where
did the photos wind up—of Reagan posing in Look five days later at the entrance to his
Malibu Ranch, leaning against a grinning lawn jockey?

Joan Quigley, one of Nancy's psychics, instructs Ronnie to swear in at midnight, Jan 2,
1967. They do it, they do it again in '81, and always, ever always the bloodbath begins.

From what I'd gathered, Nancy needed to move out
of a mansion—and fast. "But where will you go?"

I ventured, choosing an upbeat TV voice that instantly
    filled me
with regret. Nancy smiled one of her political grins.

"I'm working on it, but I could really use two
thousand to get this realtor out of my hair."

Glimmer.

LIBERACE FEB 4 1987

I swallowed my own bitter pill, paying suit
to Nancy's must-fund with generous donation,

whereupon I was gifted a spoon, with which
I began a tactful excavation of Nancy's head.

She had opened the door, of course. I'm not rude.

[Unofficial, speculative rendering of architectural floor plans for the Carmichael
Mansion. Self-drawn. Pencil and paper.
File Folder C-12.]

Feb 1967: Fake fire alarm at the governor's mansion.

Nancy deems the mansion unsafe for her children, citizens, various groups of people she
thinks about from time to time. Her favorite groups to think about are the Bloomingdales
and Jorgensens, the Tuttles and Annenbergs. Names like that.

Nancy pinpoints a furnished 6,700 square foot 6-bedroom house with a swimming pool,
pool house, and sculptured gardens. Two years later, their rich California friends buy the
house and lease it to them for $1,250 a month. Close call.

Meanwhile, in Carmichael, the Reagans build a new governor's mansion, an 8-bedroom,
8-bath 12,000 square foot home so elaborate that construction isn't finished until 1975.
When governor-elect Jerry Brown takes office, he won't live in it. No subsequent governor
will live in the house. Too gaudy. The mansion doesn't sell until 2004.

34

I noticed at once that Nancy's hairdo was
a dead giveaway, the kind of basket case that

really bites the dust when you blow holes on it.
By which I mean: each follicle, root,

and death-defying strand acquainted me
in an instant

with the euphemisms of power.

MIGUEL PIÑERO JUN 16 1988

Although she hadn't yet achieved
the hallowed grandma's nest

she would perfect in the White House,
her bob was getting

shorter and shorter
by the minute.

I thought of a stick of dynamite,
the wick burning down.

[Typed correspondence (on letterhead) from the Joffrey Ballet. Request denied 1982,
1984, 1985, 1986, 1987, 1988. File Folder G-2.]

Ron, son of Reagans, joins the senior company of the Joffrey Ballet in 1982. Nancy and
Ronald are terrified he is gay. Ron quits after one season.

Sometimes fathers never quit, son after son after son. Instead of attending eldest son
Michael's wedding on June 12, 1971, the Reagans attend the Rose Garden ceremony for
Tricia Nixon and Edward Cox.

I RE-AWAKENED   covered head-to-toe in my own grime,

phantoms or pheromones cluttering my head.

Nancy explaining the stakes of her persistent world:
"I've been sick about this contractor for weeks.

I've laughed and I've cried, I tell you,
but yesterday it dawned on me that the mansion is—"

H-A-U-N-T-E-D

I jerked hard at the shoulders, startled
by our vocal togetherness.

KLAUS NOMI AUG 6 1983

37

As she slid my stack of green across the table,
a wet substance began to bead at her scalp.

Was there a crack on the surface of her skull?
I began to worry what fissures foreshadow.

Moral bankruptcy? Itself seeming to spring.
Faith? The ploy is what you make of it.

"Bless you, child," Nancy oozed.
"Ronnie and I really value your

In a 1983 promotional photograph [framed, gift from F. LL.], Nancy drapes herself over the lap of Mr. T, who is dressed as Santa Claus.

Before he is "discovered" by Sylvester Stallone, Mr. T works as a bodyguard for A-list celebrities including Diana Ross. Mr. T's aesthetic is encoded with history.

The gold chains are a symbol that reminds me of my great African ancestors, who were brought over here as slaves with iron chains on their ankles, their wrists, their necks and sometimes around their waists... I am still a slave, only my price tag is higher.

Support arrived from distinct corners of the globe,
pouring in at first through a cascade of homosexual

anguish similar to its root force: preservation.
As self-made protective shields

expanded around us, we became dimly aware of
small villages on the outskirts of us.

Villages founded in endings and care.

["Raided Premises, by order of the..." Sign with string.
File Folder C-6.]

In 1969 St. Louis teenager Robert Rayford dies and no one can figure out what's wrong. It's disgusting, the way the doctors discuss their puzzled confrontation about his mystery illness. Eighteen years later, his DNA is brought out of cold storage and sent to molecular biologists across the country.

In May of 1969 cops kill Cal student James Rector at a rally for The People's Park in Berkeley, CA. Governor Ronald Reagan sends the National Guard to UC Berkeley to break up the protests, outfitting 2,200 troops in riot gear. Everyone gets hurt; 123 are hospitalized. Ronnie warns, enraged: *if it takes a bloodbath, let's get it over with.*

Even riots can be occupied: in June 2015 the Stonewall Inn (Riot: June 1969) is recognized as an official landmark in NYC, in 2016 a national monument.

Our way of uniting was familial, if such can
be said of a tribe of wild animals.

I paid the bill as was customary in those days.
Then Nancy took my hand again in hers, the glove,

and before long we were in the hills.

JANET SPEAKS

•

Carrying my heart on my tongue I say things openly

like I myself would be Michael working to be Janet

Janet could be Michael

Despite biological facts and Billie Jean reactions

I focus on Spiritual Education

and The Reunion of Twin

Because what I am showing here

the pre-twin development

Is How and Why Twin Flames' Souls Reunite

One time my sister & me competed in BOYS CATEGORY

like a literal hunt going on where Guys would lose

We are calm about it now

Careful not to let some energy vampires mislead us on our
soul journey

We're sending out a Major Love Ray to each
contemporary environment

and we understand them from a new perspective of compassion

We've updated twin structures for consolation

Our inner soul magnet has made supplication a functional appeal

ALL WE ARE is ONE TWIN SOUL

ONE SOUL WITH TWINS IN IT

We were always the same just as ready

in our Mirror is the root reason why

the urge to define who is a Karmic Soul Mate and who is real

Became together a complete pre-birth decided life plan

The relationship between music and movement is kinetic time

Additionally twin souls Look & Smile ALIKE

his channeling of ME & MY LOOKS reverse Michael Jackson

turning into his feminine Twin Soul their songs a

metamorphosis with me is history no going back

from the Soul Feeling I picked up clearly like with nobody

The white lines dictate floor   the figure
                          the meaning of the face

For the first time I feel A Consciousness Merging

& the different layers of the mind

Carrying my heart on my tongue I say things openly

songs sometimes or interludes or just a few words

to help other Twin Flames understand

the cruel Twist of hope to denial

when Michael sings you're just another part of me

Yes he means on a personal basis me, his other half of his soul

but he implies too the violence of family

Exposing the theater of the shoot-out made visible

the way the West becomes present, a president

suspension and the loop, how ghost becomes host

But now people, all kinds of Billie Jeans, are imitating exactly

beginning their commentary dissecting intuitive public

TWIN FLAME INTERFERENCE AND ATTACKS

With Real Science now involved my motivation is pure

In the deepest ways possible he never did anything wrong

with Children as the false accusers claimed

during his Dangerous tour

Carrying my tongue in my heart I beg you to relieve the memory

where similarity intervenes thorny and thin the way we see

with wigs is video Analysis white charcoal type

So bizarrely familiar each music video and the news announce

the arrival of the twin soul flame the noxious golden coins

in the belly

his own words and works 777 Archangel Michael

If I have to completely take on all pain

as a pile you've been struck by

the end of reward and judgment you threw Michael, too,

A second time, then

I will do so and not complain anymore

shamelessly revealing our insides

I am the twin of him and must

go strong, keep moving

if I die forget burial

just drop my body

so it can be studied

so

I can remember

MY OWN PRIVATE PARADOX

•

As we took tea in the East Wing,
Nancy told me that Rock

had AIDS and was
trying to reach her.

She said a journalist undercover as a landscaper
had pushed her to divulge secrets in the Rose Garden.

"I feel so violated," she said, pulling her long skirt
across her shins. She blinked into the sun like a cat.

COOKIE MUELLER NOV 10 1989

"I would have handed this to Ronnie, but
he was in California on Saturday

and I just couldn't endure a phone call."
"Do you think it could be true?" I asked.

As a rule, I was perpetually scandalized in the East Wing.
"I just feel so unsure," Nancy tugged at her skirt as if

it belonged to her mother, the eager beaver divorcée,
Edith "Lucky" Luckett. About whom Nancy lied:

"Mother was *feezing* cold." She insisted these odd
pronunciations

were evidence of a unique linguistic mélange

of her mother's antebellum elegance with a grit
learned during Nancy's so-called studio days.

[Phyllis Gates with Bob Thomas. *My Husband, Rock Hudson.*
Trash.]

May 1984 Rock Hudson attends a state dinner at the White House and is seated at
Nancy's table.

June 1984 a biopsy tests positive for Kaposi's sarcoma.

July 1985 Rock Hudson collapses in France, where he is seeking care for AIDS from a
renowned French military doctor. The doctor won't see him so a telegram is sent to the
White House asking if the Reagans can intervene on his behalf. Nancy Reagan denies
the request. A staffer sends the official response.

A MEMORY   I once heard Nancy flirting
with a diplomat from Belgrade,

"I'm Southern and that's what's cute about it."

I'd never tell her but actually the cute part
was that she thought no one knew about her

sleeping around in Manhattan. Or that she was
remembered as the blow job queen of Hollywood.

[Mail order type copy of J. G. Ballard, "Why I Want to Fuck Ronald Reagan."
1980 Republican National Convention.]

On August 3, 1981 the Professional Air Traffic Controllers Organization goes on strike.
President Reagan gives employees 48 hours to return to work, fires 11,345 employees
who do not return to work after the threat, and bans the strikers from federal service
for life.

Whereas I doubt she'd ever pulled on a crew knit
sweater at four in the morning, not knowing where

the light switch was, I was proof positive she knew
her way around a boatyard. Whether vice raid or

our banal cold war, we were each fluent in sailor speak.
Who had gone rogue was no matter,

impossible to distinguish her fortified apologetics
from my own myopic counterstrikes.

["Apartheid = Genocide" pins.
Box Bin 2.]

1984 Recent Nobel Prize winner Desmond Tutu travels to the US, vilifying the Reagan
administration's policy on South Africa as "immoral, evil and totally un-Christian."

Reagan's response? *"It is counterproductive for one country to splash itself all over the
headlines, demanding that another government do something."*

1984-86 anti-apartheid protests erupt across the United States, where organizing at
hundreds of universities and colleges succeeds in mass divestment from companies in
business with South Africa.

September 26, 1986, Reagan vetoes The Comprehensive Anti-Apartheid Act, a bill
passed by Congress calling for far-reaching sanctions against South Africa's racist
regime. The following month the Senate votes 78-21 to override his veto.

In response to some perceived empathy
from me, Nancy continued, "Thank you for caring."

She came at me in sections.
To deflect, I dug up an old memory, recounting

every detail from the dressing room in Uniondale.
I could refer to that night

as a low point of my emotional life,

but, as I've become more generous with my "past selves"
(as Liz likes to say), I simply study this moment as a

kind of Zen koan. My own private paradox.

[Paul Vitello. "David Jones, Florist to Hollywood, Dead at 78." Newsprint.
File Folder J-11.]

Nancy never pays for anything. Tight as a drum. Even in later years, she salutes the name
of her florist up a flagpole: David Jones. When people send her flowers, her chosen
florist banks the orders as credit in Nancy's account rather than delivering. Whenever she
needs to send flowers, Nancy just *picks up the phone and sings.* All free; a heist.

I'd agreed to sing a song. "Just one song once,"
I'd brazenly told my agent.

DiLeo, that ambitious little Druid, arranged me
for the benefit at Astor Place for Oscar Wilde.

Unless it was the show this century at Carnegie Hall.
Or, Eddie Murphy in a car, with me?

How can I remember after so much violence?
For my blameless confusion, DiLeo

slapped me, popping me in the face with a fist
the size of the quid pro quo he was handing over.

VICTOR HUGO ROJAS 1993

Sixteen minutes later,

I wrapped dark sunglasses in a tidy bow around my face.
My head so heavy I could only turn in

slow motion, like a bus. Clutching microphone
in hand, I was flung onto the stage, a bowl full of

weighted fruit on the balance, where each vowel
became a message. The holes were instant.

My voice lifted suffering to fill them.

ESSEX HEMPHILL NOV 4 1995

Nancy's eyes rolled back into her head in such a way
that I was reminded, tenderly, of Hamlet.

Of course I knew what to do.

I'd have to crawl out of my skin
to find out what was killing them.

MARIO COOPER MAY 29 2015

IRRESISTIBLE FORCES

•

On February 20, 1987, the Japanese entertainment company Konami released the run and gun video arcade game *Contra*.

Content-wise, the game remixes 1980's popular media. Released as *Gryzor* in Europe, *Contra*'s cover art is based on Arnold Schwarzenegger as "Dutch" in the 1987 film *Predator*.

Into the 1990's and early 2000's, *Contra* remained a popular series, spawning sequels and imitators that could be played across gaming platforms.

On November 13, 1986, President Reagan addressed the public on national television to acknowledge weapon transfers to Iran. He asserted that the United States had not traded arms for hostages.

In fact, the smuggling of weapons, mostly missiles, had begun in August 1985.

Hezbollah was holding seven United States citizens hostage in Lebanon.

Because Iran was under an arms embargo, the weapons were smuggled through Israel.

Part of the profit from these sales went to fund the Contras in Nicaragua, the right-wing, anti-Sandinista group backed by the C.I.A.

The funding of the Contras was prohibited by the Boland Amendment, which was passed by Congress 1982-1984. The illicit sale of arms to Iran occurred for at least fourteen months.

PLAYER 1

The Konami Code is a cheat entered at the start of a video game.

When the title screen appears, the player presses a series of buttons to unleash a prize.

In *Contra*, the Konami Code grants the player thirty lives instead of three.

PLAYER 2

On March 4, 1987, President Reagan addressed the public once again, this time to take "full responsibility" for his actions in the trading of arms for hostages.

Investigations by Congress and the Reagan-appointed Tower Commission resulted in fourteen indictments and eleven convictions, most of which were overturned through appeal. No one served time.

In the final days of George H. W. Bush's presidency, all remaining men involved in the Iran-Contra scandal were pardoned. Bush had served as Vice President throughout the Reagan administration. He denied knowledge of the scandal throughout his campaign and administration, although evidence suggests that he knew the details of the exchanges at the time.

Konami's *Contra* features two characters. Bill is a blonde who wears a white tank top and a blue bandana. Lance is shirtless with dark hair in a red bandana.

Bill and Lance are Warholian babes: Joe D'Allesandro on steroids; Elvis with a gun.

The game's primary innovation is the *Contra* jump.

When the player presses "A," the fighters curl into somersaults and spin through the air.

The Revolución Popular Sandinista was the result of ten years of grassroots organizing. The FSLN (Sandinista National Liberation Front) was founded in 1961 by student activists in Managua. In 1978-79, the FSLN overthrew the Somocista regime, a dynasty that began in 1936.

The revolution ushered in huge economic, agrarian, and cultural reform that would rebuild Nicaraguan society from the ruins left by dictatorship and war.

Money poured in from the Cold War superpowers. Nicaragua received $80 million in aid from the Carter Administration in 1979. Upon his inauguration, Reagan cut off all aid, condemning the Sandinista government for sending arms to rebels in El Salvador.

Soon enough, opposition forces united against the new government and became known as Contras. They received immense financial and military support from the United States, including arms, military training, and the covert backing of human rights violations and the killing/disappearing of civilians.

USE MEMORY EDITING OR THE FOLLOWING CHEAT CODES

IDKFA
RICHTER
BIGDADDY
MAPWARP
GODMODE
BLOODCODE

FOR

UNLIMITED BULLET TIME
INFINTE 1-UPS
UNLOCK FANTASY ZONE
LEVEL SELECT
DEBUG
ALWAYS BE ON FIRE

62

In the game, Bill and Lance lead an elite task force that specializes in guerrilla warfare. Bill and Lance have been deployed to an island near New Zealand, where they must destroy enemy forces controlled by an unknowable alien entity.

The game's concluding theme is titled "Sandinistas."

The Revolución Popular Sandinista remains one of the most significant experiments in socialist democracy.

In the summer of 1980 the new government began the Nicaraguan Literacy Campaign, a now iconic literacy program that was awarded the UNESCO Literacy Award. It was estimated that half of the people of Nicaragua could not read.

As with much of the organizing and strategies of the FSLN, the program was modeled on the Cuban Literacy Program, which raised literacy rates in Cuba to 96% within two years following the revolution.

NICARAGUA DEBE SOBREVIVIR

ID Number: 3858
Maker: Asociación de Mujeres Nicaragüenses Luisa Amanda Espinoza; Orlando Valenzuela
Technique: offset
Date Made: Circa 1985
Place Made: Central America: Nicaragua
Measurements: 23.5 x 17 in.; 60 x 43 cm
Main Subject: Nicaragua; women
Materials: paper (fiber product); wrapped, corners
Digitized: Y

Full Text: Nicaragua Debe Sobrevivir Nicaragua Must Survive AMNLAE

Acquisition Number: 1996-132
Notes: Orlando Valenzuela's Miliciana de Waswalito (1984) is a photograph taken in Matagalpa, Nicaragua.

63

Multiplayer video games revolutionized the social potential of gaming.

In early iterations, interaction was scripted as partnership, competition, or rivalry.

Within this framework, Bill and Lance function as partners—a homosocial co-op bent on destroying the feminine Other.

Exhibition Annotation:

Soon after the 1979 overthrow of the U.S. backed Somoza dictatorship in Nicaragua by the Sandinista National Liberation Front (FSLN), the Reagan administration formed a mercenary army called the Contras (Counter-Revolutionaries), to destroy the schools, health clinics and agricultural cooperatives supported by the FSLN. This poster of a Sandinista militia member nursing her child was widely reproduced internationally. It was prominent in the "Let Nicaragua Live" campaign to send construction materials, school supplies, seeds tools and medical equipment to Nicaragua in the 1980s, to help counter the destruction caused by the Contras. The Sandinista Revolution was marked by an unprecedented level of women's participation. By 1987, it was reported that 67% of active members in the popular militia and 80% of guards—an estimated 50,000 nationwide—were women.

PLAYER 2

By the 1980's, enrollment in and violence between Bloods and Crips had escalated in the United States, primarily due to drastic unemployment and the introduction of crack cocaine to urban streets, facilitated through the C.I.A.'s funding of drug cartels.

In *Contra*, levels alternate between side-scrolling play and three point perspective.

Players fight an incessant stream of enemies as they navigate passageways and destroy sensors on their way toward the enemy's last line of defense.

Backronyms for the name Crips include "Common Revolution in Progress" and "Community Resources for Independent People."

Written on the heels of the 1992 Watts Truce (a peace agreement negotiated between rival groups), the Bloods/Crips Proposal envisioned a radical future for Los Angeles. The Proposal outlined the rebuilding of communities through funding for healthcare, educational, and rejuvenation programs. The Proposal held that if their list of demands was met, they would rid the streets of drug dealers and match funds for an HIV/AIDS awareness center to be operated by a staff of people of color.

PLAYER 1

According to the rules of the game, players lose a life if Bill or Lance is touched by an enemy or bullet.

"I never injure people, but only make them afraid."
Shi Nai'an, 水滸傳

PLAYER 2

The Reagan administration's support of the Contras was funded through the illegal smuggling of crack cocaine from Nicaragua to Los Angeles.

At his 1996 trial, "Freeway" Rick Ross's lawyers claimed the crack he sold came from the C.I.A.

Ross had been captured through a set-up involving the Nicaraguan drug lord who was also Ross's main source, Oscar Danilo Blandón.

Blandón had served as the primary connect between the C.I.A. and the Contras during the Iran-Contra affair.

Ross served over ten years in prison.

Blandón served two.

PLAYER 1

Due to the graphic limitations of the original Nintendo Entertainment System, Bill and Lance lost their individual character designs and became shirtless clones, distinguishable by blue pants (Player 1) and red pants (Player 2).

PLAYER 2

Despite
Oliver
media
as if we
President
arms

souls. And then bring it all up and out. To where we are now.

remember. Look into those files we keep in our bodies and

history, but inside. It makes one go deep inside, go back and

NORA MISELEM: It's like traveling the length of one's own

bad. Or made you feel good. Or if it's been the same for both.

talking like this, has been difficult for you. If it's made you feel

MARGARET RANDALL: I was going to ask if this interview, if

firsthand testimony by
North and others, the
still presents the scandal
may never know whether
Reagan was aware of these
sales.

PLAYER 1

In a 2002 sequel, *Contra: Shattered Soldier*, Bill and Lance are enemies.

At the start of the game, Bill is released from cryogenic prison, where he was serving a sentence of 10,000 years for accidentally destroying 80% of the Earth's population.

Although formerly assumed dead by Bill's hand, Lance—it is revealed— has in the years since merged with an alien cell and become the commander of the terrorist organization known as Blood Falcon.

1980-1993 Funding for federal employment and training programs is cut in half

1986 Anti-Drug Abuse Act passes in the Senate (97-2 vote) and House (392-16) 100-to-1 longer prison sentences for crack vs. powder cocaine increased mandatory minimum sentencing

PLAYER 2

The Office of Public Diplomacy was a covert program formed under Reagan that reported directly to Oliver North.

The intra-agency office strategized with the C.I.A. and Army intelligence to disseminate what it dubbed "white propaganda," false news stories intended to sway public opinion against the Sandinistas.

1986 the first HIV criminalization laws are passed most laws criminalize non-disclosure most people believed any intimate contact could put one at risk

1990 the Ryan White Care Act passes in Congress requires states to demonstrate the "ability to prosecute intentional transmission" in order to receive funding statutes increase sentences for sex workers and may include acts that do not transmit HIV (such as spitting) these early HIV laws are still used to prosecute

1980-1993 Spending on prison industrial complex increases 521%

PLAYER 1

In these games, the fear of femininity is so entrenched that the repression of this fear materializes in gorgeous biological and mythical forms.

PLAYER 2

Nancy Reagan's favorite flower is the peony, a traditional floral symbol of China that has 33 species.

Ukiyo-e artist Utagawa Kuniyoshi (1798-1861) is a Japanese master most remembered for his illustrations of the classic Chinese novel 水滸傳, often translated as *Water Margin*, *Outlaws of the Marsh*, or *All Men Are Brothers*. The Japanese translation is *Suikoden*.

水滸傳 is an epic about 108 rebels who fight for and protect the common people.

From 1827-1830, Kuniyoshi painted tattooed warrior-heroes in kinetic portraits. Many of the tattoos feature peonies.

In his series, the peony functions as a masculine motif associated with a disregard for consequence.

African Americans are incarcerated in state prisons at a rate that is 5.1 times the imprisonment of whites. In five states (Iowa, Minnesota, New Jersey, Vermont, and Wisconsin), the disparity is more than 10 to 1.

In twelve states, more than half of the prison population is black: Alabama, Delaware, Georgia, Illinois, Louisiana, Maryland, Michigan, Mississippi, New Jersey, North Carolina, South Carolina, and Virginia. Maryland, whose prison population is 72% African American, tops the nation.

In eleven states, at least 1 in 20 adult black males is in prison.

In Oklahoma, the state with the highest overall black incarceration rate, 1 in 15 black males of ages 18 and older is in prison.

States exhibit substantial variation in the range of racial disparity, from a black/white ratio of 12.2:1 in New Jersey to 2.4:1 in Hawaii.

Latinos are imprisoned at a rate that is 1.4 times the rate of whites. Hispanic/white ethnic disparities are particularly high in states such as Massachusetts (4.3:1), Connecticut (3.9:1), Pennsylvania (3.3:1), and New York (3.1:1).

"The Color of Justice: Racial and Ethnic Disparity in State Prisons" (2016)
Ashley Nellis, Ph.D, The Sentencing Project

PLAYER 1

In psychology, disregard for consequence is called *moral disengagement*, a complex process whereby moral reaction is separated from inhuman action in order to reframe destructive behavior as morally acceptable.

PLAYER 2

The Japanese entertainment company Konami released a role-playing video game called *Suikoden* in 1998.

The game's plot is loosely based on the novel, and the player can recruit up to 108 allies to fight a string of political battles against Empire.

PLAYER 1

In Chinese mythology, Bai Mudan (White Peony) is a beautiful courtesan famous for her humiliating seductions of men.

"Dora Maria

the warrior girl

who blasted the tyrant's

heart"

PLAYER 2

Daisy Zamora

There are no established traditions for a First Lady's funeral.

PLAYER 1

In some versions of her story, Bai Mudan becomes immortal; in others, she has a heart of gold. In the opera *Lü Dongbin and Bai Mudan*, she is no longer a powerful courtesan. She is the daughter of a man who owns a drugstore.

PLAYER 2

For her March 11, 2016 funeral at the Ronald Reagan Presidential Library in Simi Valley, California, every detail is planned and arranged in advance by Nancy Reagan herself.

Her casket is covered in white peonies.

PRAYER 1

To win the game the player must

kill the head of the alien that
spawns deadly larvae from its mouth

(the feminine)

kill the giant beating heart that
grows from cracks in the ancient wall

(the feminine in the self)

PRAYER 2

The words that scroll down

the final screen of *Contra* are

CONSIDER YOURSELF A HERO.
CONSIDER YOURSELF A HERO.
CONSIDER YOURSELF A HERO.
CONSIDER YOURSELF A HERO.
CONSIDER YOURSELF A HERO.
CONSIDER YOURSELF A HERO.

U.S. military assistance to right-wing death squads was justified through recycled Cold War rhetoric vilifying "Marxist guerrillas" and stoking fears about the spread of communism. Reagan heralded the Contras as freedom fighters, as he did with the mujahideen in Afghanistan.

Reagan's shoot 'em up policies backed by capital and the flagrant disregard of international law resulted in

20,000+
dead in
Nicaragua
70,000+
dead in
El Salvador
200+
disappeared in
Honduras
200,000+
dead in Guatemala

In 1986, the International Court of Justice rules in favor of Nicaragua and against the United States, awarding $17 billion in damages. The United States refuses to take part in the trial and successfully blocks payment of the reparations through its ties in the United Nations.

Between 1980-1990 the number of incarcerated people increased 142%

incarcerated populations doubled at federal, state, and local jail levels

1980: 41,000 incarcerated for drug crimes
2014: 488,400 incarcerated for drug crimes

...$3 billion, C.I.A.'s covert funding to Afghanistan, 1981-1989...

...$8.5 million arms package sold to Saudi Arabia in 1981...

...over $10 million in military shipments to Guatemala 1982-1983...

Box Office Report

Terminator (1984)	$78,371,200
Aliens (1986)	$131,060,248
Predator (1987)	$98,267,558
Die Hard (1988)	$140,767,956

JUST SAY AIDS

•

She told me not to shave. "What's the point
of shaving?" Nancy asked with outstanding

rhetorical frustration. We were watching a film
and eating delicious bonbon spinach morsels

the White House chef made for her. Special her.

Convinced that my propensity for hairlessness was
a waste of energy, Nancy nagged me in perpetuity.

SISTER FLORENCE NIGHTMARE AUG 15 1984

We were on a kick with popular movies
featuring water and took turns choosing films.

This secret sport of ours is how I discovered
everything Nancy thought she knew about blondes.

Naturally, I'd selected *Splash* (1984),
which I'd been obsessively watching for weeks.

MARLON RIGGS APR 5 1994

Of course the claim that my pores did not produce
facial hair couldn't cut mustard with Nancy.

She'd be off on one of her monologues: "It seems to me
that not shaving is one of the biggest perks of manhood…"

As if to taunt me, if only

worn down with attitude

so as to peel me, weekly

SAM D'ALLESANDRO FEB 3 1988

I had presented the film as a modern-day adaptation lifted
from Ovid's *Metamorphoses*, but Nancy wouldn't hear of it.

She chose to process her feelings about Daryl
over top the always-screaming soundtrack.

JOBRIATH AUG 4 1983

As I was saying, Daryl Hannah was a troubling figure
for Nancy—she had a cathartic struggle with blondes

her entire life—but on this particular day I must stop
and reflect on what was ultimately a morbid fascination

with Daryl Hannah's "bohemianism." For that's what
Nancy saw in her, and Nancy loathed

bohemianism with hatred
she normally reserved for drug addicts.

[Closet, never washed.]

I remember his face when I bought it. A "Just Say No" shirt, light wear, near perfect
condition but for the bleach stain near the No. He thought it was funny.

I assured him, it was not.

Daryl was a blonde where Nancy
and I could agree to disagree,

which was the most common ground
I believe we ever shared.

The reason Nancy and I enjoyed spending time together
was not about getting along. Truth be told, the only person

she ever liked was Frank Sinatra. In my practical opinion
Frank was an inconsequential warrior-songbird,

her cat in a paper bag. All wail, no backbone. Nancy
merely had to give it a shake and he'd come out to play.

DONDI OCT 2 1998

That the heavy hand of destiny controlled
her life too is what made Daryl Hannah

as the mermaid Madison an attractive figure for us.
Where we disagreed was the tail—and to a lesser degree,

the casting of Tom Hanks. Predictably, Nancy adored
him. In the film, Madison's rubbery tail is scalloped

faux mermaid skin reminiscent of blood oranges
burnt to a crisp, or ye olde tongue of plastic brûlée.

Dealer's choice.

Something fitting

something twinning

unadulterated cerulean potential

KIYOSHI KUROMIYA MAY 10 2000

Understandably, there was a shared charisma between Tom Hanks's hair and the wild viscosity of Madison's tail.

[Nothing. Nowhere.]

Beginning in 1982, each time AIDS is mentioned in the White House Press Briefing Room, press secretary Larry Speakes feigns ignorance while cracking gay sex jokes.

It's not until September 17, 1985 that Reagan mentions AIDS publicly. His first speech on AIDS isn't until May 31, 1987.

A RECOGNITION   That the tail is indescribable I'll assume

is already known, but the aura itself—

"of the tail" as they say—is something to behold,
over and over again, to behold.

[Geraldine Ferraro America's 1ˢᵗ Woman VP button, heart-shaped.
Convention vendor, Box Bin 2.

"Just Say AIDS" T-shirt 1991, same box.]

In 1984, the Democratic National Convention convenes in San Francisco, where 100,000 activists march from the Castro to the Moscone Center to demand funding for AIDS research.

In 1986, Reagan intimate William F. Buckley writes for mandatory testing, segregation, and tattooing of HIV+ status in the *New York Times*.

At the 1986 rededication of the Statue of Liberty, the Reagans laugh on camera at an especially crude homophobic joke made by Bob Hope. Visiting heads of state from France are appalled.

Nancy was nearly silent on the subject, no matter my curse.

"It's so life-like," she'd exclaim like clockwork each time
the tail hit the linoleum on its way out of the tub.

"But Nancy, it's so much *more* than that!" I'd urge.
If only I could find a track for her dialogue to travel.

"It's just so life-like," she'd slowly gasp. Nancy certainly
had an appreciation for the life-like part of life.

Confrontation with the real often slowed
her down to about quarter speed.

I corrected, unheard as always,
"Nancy, it's technically limb-like."

PAUL THEK AUG 10 1988

By this point, she'd drifted into a world of her own
while I skipped trivial prophesies off the cold surface

of our meeting. (e.g., "In the next scene that tail's
gonna cry for mercy like the Keating

Five at a poker table!") The thing with Nancy
was that she never heeded my warnings.

[Newspaper clipping, A-5.
File Folder E 1-10.]

On March 31, 1981 John Hinckley, Jr. attempts to assassinate Ronald Reagan. Three
months later, the New York Times runs an article titled "Rare Cancer Seen in 41
Homosexuals." Nancy, codename RAINBOW, has to fight to be allowed to enter the
emergency room where Ronald, codename RAWHIDE, is fighting for his life.

They don't know how it is with us, he has to know I'm here.

The question on everyone's lips: Who knows why the Reagans receive the gayest
codenames in Presidential history?

In March 2013 the historic Chelsea leather bar RAWHIDE closes when rent nearly
doubles, $15,000 to $27,000 a month. Inside are Herb Ritts posters, Tom of Finland
prints, and Michael Jackson on the jukebox singing "Smooth Criminal."

Just as Ron could never fasten her clasps, Nancy strung
her own beads and it just so happened that Tom Hanks

was one tune she could sing. Otherwise, she was
tone deaf, with a neurosurgeon for a stepfather.

If *Splash* was the best of times, I began to suspect
that the worst would mean a sea of death.

[Gran Fury, *AIDSGATE*. Print, 1987.
File Folder E-15.]

Finally in 1987, Reagan offers his first major speech on AIDS. During the Reagan
administration, 116,000 people are diagnosed with AIDS and 70,000 die. That
same month, Gran Fury mounts "Let the Record Show" in a New Museum window, an
installation in cardboard and neon depicting six Americans (including Reagan, Jerry
Falwell, William F. Buckley, Jesse Helms, and Cory SerVaas) as war criminals.

In 1990, the year AIDS deaths in the US pass 100,000, Reagan apologizes for his
neglect during the epidemic. In 1994, Benetton runs an ad designed by Oliviero Toscani
depicting Reagan with KS lesions.

I was terrified, but I soon realized Nancy
was asleep, exhausted by our mermaid.

On my way out, I scrawled a note
on the pad near the telephone:

Dear Nancy, Love Michael.

I hopped down the steps and swaggered to the bus stop
as if my tail were a thousand yards long.

SWORN TO SECRECY

•

At this point, Nancy Reagan was
eating mango out of my hands

between crying jags.

I spun an evocative tale about three men in a tube
that soon had her laughing through the tears like

an old-fashioned barrel roll.
You know, a butcher and a baker.

[White House Recipe Card.
Kitchen.]

The White House recipe for Onion Wine Soup appears a bit heavy on cream for my
taste. I've learned to let mine simmer for seven minutes rather than five as the recipe calls.

In 1989, the IRS began an investigation prompted by Nancy's failure to disclose gowns
and jewelry gifted to her throughout the administration. Although she vowed, in 1982, to
return all borrowed items, she fell back on old ways, surrounding herself with Galanos,
Adolfo, Bill Blass, Bulgari.

The IRS determined in 1992 that the Reagans had failed to disclose fashion items that
totaled at least three million dollars.

I preserve the recipe card (Signed) in my copy of Close to the Knives (unsigned, 1991),
which I keep on the shelf with my cookbooks. And the decorative miniature fishes I found
near the pier.

"Oh, Julie," into my eyes Nancy laughed—
inexplicably, that's what she called me.

These instances of mistaken identity were
off-limits for me. I couldn't bring myself to

enter a cave that everyone denied existed, so I wandered
from two directions: Did she even know who I was?

Did she know somcone else? Or who I might become?

Nancy clasped hands as if we were women in mourning.
I shook my head and began to play up the scene.

GIA CARANGI NOV 18 1986

I suggested Nancy's bigotry toward Daryl was
at root reflective of, one, a nascent confusion

with the history of Europe, and, two, an ill-timed and
unfortunate—likely repressed—encounter with sea life.

Did she know the difference between bolsheviks and bohemians?

I couldn't actually defend Daryl, who I admired
because she brought out the schoolboy in me.

I knew a suspected breach in loyalty on this point
would drive Nancy to unmitigated fury.

BILL OLANDER MAR 18 1989

Nancy reveled in performing her own distaste,
but to me this rage looked more like envy,

an infatuation with her opposition.
If I were more contemporary, I'd call it

cathecting with the light on but the psychoanalytic
never held much purchase for me,

apart from sheer audacity,
its magic.

JEROME CAJA NOV 3 1995

A descendent of Ovid, Freud could turn
worlds too with the slightest hands.

Like mine, I mused, looking over the digits
I thought of as my own girlish tendrils.

I had always wanted to understand these unspoken wars
and romances between women, which is why I'd learned

to steer Nancy's anger around like a bus.
(I'd once tried to drive a bus when I was

in Atlanta performing with my brothers, so
I know how difficult they can be to turn.)

The lone photograph [Framed, 1990] I possess of Joan Quigley, Nancy's astrologer, is worn with elements. It must have gotten wet—a flood, perhaps, or merely rain, a glass of water. Whatever it was this contamination enhances the photograph's aura.

Joan's on the phone with two astrological charts spread before her; right hand prone on the table holding tortoise shell spectacles. She appears to be sleeping, two eyelids closed studying the charts: a mask at work.

Imagine me skipper of Nancy's bullhorns,
one hand on each, and her snorting smoke.

I flipped Nancy's blonde switch
without regard for the aftermath.

I yawned, "Has *she* ever been to the White House?"

TSENG KWONG CHI MAR 10 1990

The conspiracy theorist in me quite genuinely would
have loved to know, but having planted a future

nightmare in Nancy's head, I found myself
overtaken with the desire to offer my shoulder to her

by any means necessary.

KUWASI BALAGOON DEC 13 1986

I whispered a string of secret cruelties
that soared like dark arrows at my target:

a strangely medieval version of Ms. Hannah.

For Nancy's sake, I dragged the entirety
of my imagination for petty fictions that

might rebuild the wall around her crusading heart.

Once I got myself into a rhythm, I was able to
automate my storytelling so that I could figure

a larger mystery at the corner of the scene.

For I had begun to feel the slight
pang of heartbroken news.

B. MICHAEL HUNTER JAN 23 2001

I glimpsed the sad VHS case, open on the table
beside the controls for the sound system.

Out of the foreground of my eye,
I felt I had something to hide.

An open trap;

a shell case of misery—

How would I manage the failure of my last ditch
attempt at throwing Nancy overboard?

Through muffled sighs and frequent jabs for breath,
Nancy continued to refer to me as "Julie."

In my panic I sorted through my imaginary
Rolodex of films in search of a key, a sign.

A reclusive outer bank with the promise of shade.

ANGIE XTRAVAGANZA MAR 31 1993

That's when I heard it, a lisp on a cup:
the perennial wake of the diver's splash.

AMERICA'S BRAIN

•

a play in diorama

<u>Characters</u>
BABY ROSS is 15.
Other characters are perfectly dressed, age 25.

Scene I
Domestic space where glamour reigns.

DIANA ROSS

I simply won't. I won't, Evan!

BABY ROSS

But Mother, it's my choice. My career.

DIANA ROSS

I simply won't have you camping around with a cigarette in your hand.
Even *if* it's the best role of your life!

BABY ROSS

Mom, I honestly thought you would be happy for me.

DIANA ROSS

Chin up, darling! Up! Come to mommy.

Now, Evan, baby, I WILL NOT have you smoking on screen, no matter how dying-of-AIDS this character is.

Can you feel this? I'm pressing into your spleen right now.

BABY ROSS

But why??

DIANA ROSS

Because that's where actors keep their acting juice!

BABY ROSS

Mom. Where in the world did you get that idea?

DIANA ROSS

From Nancy Reagan, the Hollywood High Queen!

BABY ROSS

Who's that?

Scene 2

Casting call for Queen Latifah's critically acclaimed film Life Support *also starring Anna Deavere Smith and Tracee Ellis Ross.*

TRACEE ELLIS ROSS

Mother told Evan that playing a man with HIV who smokes would be dangerous. She warned him.

ANNA DEAVERE SMITH

Sometimes a warning isn't enough.

TRACEE ELLIS ROSS

I'm so sick of waiting around in this damned hospital.

ANNA DEAVERE SMITH

Hospital? I thought this was a scientific lab!

QUEEN LATIFAH

Welcome, ladies, to the set of *Donovan's Brain*, the 1953 sci-fi film starring a young Nancy Reagan.

TRACEE ELLIS ROSS

Doctor, Doctor! Do you have a diagnosis? Will this brain live?

QUEEN LATIFAH

Sadly, no. But if I've learned one thing in this career, ladies, it is to *never* give up hope on the brain. Think of this organ of ours as an alien... Brains can do almost anything.

TRACEE ELLIS ROSS

Well, they can't take over our minds, can they?

ANNA DEAVERE SMITH
Brains don't do mind control, people do mind control!

NANCY REAGAN enters.

ANNA DEAVERE SMITH
Well, well, well... Who's *she*?

QUEEN LATIFAH
That's Nancy Reagan, former MGM star turned First Lady of
Sacramento turned Joan Didion's punching bag turned First Lady who
turned out Frank Sinatra!

ANNA DEAVERE SMITH
Damn.

QUEEN LATIFAH
Don't tell her I said that.

NANCY REAGAN
Doctor, have you figured out how to keep the brain alive in a body
ravaged by AIDS-related illness?

QUEEN LATIFAH
Excuse me?

NANCY REAGAN
I have asked you on more than one occasion to *solve AIDS* with this
magic brain. Can you imagine what it took for me to find and secure a
pure brain of the 1950's? I had to call in a special favor from my dear
old stepdad, Loyal Davis, neurosurgeon to the stars.

QUEEN LATIFAH
Wait, you know a real neurosurgeon? Why am I even here?

NANCY REAGAN

Why are you arguing with me when you should be finding something
for us to say to gay people like yourself such as my beloved hairdresser,
Mr. Julius.

MR. JULIUS

Happy Hairdresser, Happy Nancy!

QUEEN LATIFAH

What is there to say that you haven't not said already?

BABY ROSS

Mrs. Reagan, my mother told me you are a famous actress, and I just
love famous actresses.

NANCY REAGAN

Come along with me, you smart little boy.

BABY ROSS

Mom, can I?

DIANA ROSS is in shock? Is winning? Is hurt?

NANCY REAGAN

As a matter of fact, young man, my first role was in a 1940 educational
video about polio called "National Foundation for Infantile Paralysis."
I played *A Volunteer...*

Scene 3
A black and white hospital for black and white children.
Just like the films Nancy used to make!

A VOLUNTEER

I can let you see him now.

DIANA ROSS

Oh, thank god. Thank god, he's alive!

A VOLUNTEER

Let me warn you, his brain has suffered some real indignities.

DIANA ROSS

Not internally, I hope?

A VOLUNTEER

No. All external wounds dealt by a world unaccustomed to sex.

BABY ROSS

Mother, is that you?

A VOLUNTEER

No, hon, I'm Nancy Reagan, remember? The woman who saved you
and brought you here to survive. This— is all thanks— to me!

DIANA ROSS

Baby, have you suffered?

A VOLUNTEER

Ma'am? I hate to interrupt—but this hospital's short of Volunteers,
and you really seem to care.

                        DIANA ROSS
I'm not acting.

                        A VOLUNTEER
Yours is a decidedly regal empathy. IS IT REAL?

                        BABY ROSS
My Princess Mom.

                        A VOLUNTEER
I wonder if you could help us out. I mean in a full-time capacity.
Unpaid, the work is, but you look like a professional mourner.

                PRINCESS DIANA/DIANA ROSS
I'm in need of more mourning myself. /

                        (singing,)
Touch me in the morning.

                        BABY ROSS
Mom?

                PRINCESS DIANA/DIANA ROSS
Don't call me "Mom."

                        A VOLUNTEER
What's happening to your brain?

                        PRINCESS DIANA
I am myself. I'm simply turning into myself.

NANCY REAGAN
Oh my, you're suddenly a real princess charming!

PRINCESS DIANA
But will they let me have little princes?

NANCY REAGAN
Why not? A woman like you, blonde and British, so devastating in heels... Why can't you have the kingdom when you're the only reason the kingdom comes?

PRINCESS DIANA
I think they're afraid of me.

NANCY REAGAN laughs.

PRINCESS DIANA
I'm afraid they're afraid of me. My own royal family. Charles. The Queen. All of our friends. Oh, Nancy...

NANCY REAGAN
There, there. Why don't you come to America and reinvent yourself as an actress. Have you considered it?

PRINCESS DIANA
Impossible. They hate me. They really hate me.

NANCY REAGAN
Princess Diana, no one fears or hates strong women like us. They need us for life support.

PRINCESS DIANA
They use us to determine what is alive.

NANCY REAGAN

And what is dead.

PRINCESS DIANA

And in return, we show them where our hearts are.

NANCY REAGAN

And they destroy them.

Scene 4

The Presidential General Electric Theater Library, Scientific Lab, and Casting Couch.

RONALD REAGAN

Welcome to the General Electric Theater! This job will begin to make me rich and help me learn to simulate political aptitude.

NANCY REAGAN'S GAZE

As the public spokesman for a wholesome American company, Ronnie made lots of dough, got us tons of free kitchens, and won the hearts of millions of consumers.

RONALD REAGAN

Consumers whose brains eventually started to hear things the way I heard 'em, see things the way things should be seen, shoot whoever up the way I wanted to see 'em shooted 'em up!

NANCY REAGAN'S GAZE

The brains of millions around the world but mostly in conservative parts of the United States were beating like hearts for this old dreamboat of mine.

RONALD REAGAN

Let's go sailing!

NANCY REAGAN'S GAZE

We wanted you to say we just couldn't live without him.

RONALD REAGAN

Or horseback riding!

NANCY REAGAN'S GAZE
(to screen,)
He sure knows how to show us a good time, doesn't he?

BRAIN burps.

RONALD REAGAN
I reckon we ought to tell 'em another bedtime story, Nancy.

NANCY REAGAN'S GAZE
They're all bedtime stories, silly!

RONALD REAGAN
Hmmm. I suppose you're right. But I don't like the ones with blood.

NANCY REAGAN'S GAZE
Honey, we really should leave out the ones with blood. Or at least leave out the bloody parts!

RONALD REAGAN
We can just tell them that their experience of economics means suffering and that suffering is important.

NANCY REAGAN'S GAZE
(to camera,)
Can't you see why I fell in love with him, this ol' dreamy, brainless chump of mine with a crank machine for a heart?

RONALD REAGAN
You know me, mean old mommy. My little jellybean.

NANCY REAGAN'S GAZE
(sitting on his lap as if he were Mr. T,)
I sure do, Mr. President.

RONALD REAGAN

Why don't you slip into something sexy, something red?

NANCY REAGAN'S GAZE

Whatever suits you, Governor.

RONALD REAGAN

My red devil. Come over and put your jellybean in my mouth.

NANCY REAGAN'S GAZE

That's what I live for, baby.

RONALD REAGAN

I'm a baby Ronnie.

NANCY REAGAN'S GAZE

Bad Baby Ronnie doesn't get any jellybeans.

RONALD REAGAN

Waaaaaaah.

NANCY REAGAN'S GAZE

Do you have a poopy jellybean, Baby Ronnie?

RONALD REAGAN nods and sucks his thumb.

NANCY REAGAN inserts herself.

NANCY REAGAN

Would you like me to put my jellybean up in there, Baby Ronnie? Up
there in the dark?

RONALD REAGAN nods and sucks his thumb.

NANCY REAGAN
(screams,)
How's this feel? How does it feeeeel?

Scene 5

An American naval base in a not-American country.

NANCY REAGAN

Thank you so much for being here.

MICHAEL JACKSON

It's so nice to be wherever we are. It's really nice to be wherever with nice people on such a nice day.

NANCY REAGAN

Isn't it?

MICHAEL JACKSON

And all the nice people at Pepsi. Good to see you again. And other people I don't know, who seem to be in the Navy.

NANCY REAGAN

You are really very well behaved.

PRINCESS DIANA

We all genuinely love you, Michael. That's the thing.

> *MICHAEL smiles. His companion, BUBBLES, is nearly moved to tears.*

PRINCESS DIANA

But we're here at this secret location to talk to you.

NANCY REAGAN

To talk to you both about something important.

MICHAEL JACKSON

Is it AIDS? Because I wasn't going to do anything. Bubbles and I are just hoping to see some things.

BUBBLES gestures meaningfully.

RONALD REAGAN

What's AIDS?

NANCY REAGAN

Don't worry about it.

PRINCESS DIANA

I wouldn't go that far, Nancy.

NANCY REAGAN

Di, don't even try.

MICHAEL JACKSON

So what *do* you want to speak with me about?

PRINCESS DIANA

You see, Nancy and I have gotten ourselves into a bit of a bind.

NANCY REAGAN

We need to ask a favor of you because it's something we can't do ourselves.

PRINCESS DIANA

We don't mean to scare you with this—it's going to sound like science fiction. Nevertheless, we need you to see about a gigantic MotherHeart at the bottom of the Pacific. Not too far off the coast of California, in fact. It won't take very long.

RONALD REAGAN

Mother. Heart.

PRINCESS DIANA

That's right, Mr. President!

NANCY REAGAN

Michael, we need you to lead a team: you, Ronnie, and Bubbles. And two diving troops off this ship. There are some sensors you'll have to disable—

PRINCESS DIANA

It's not going to be easy, in other words.

MICHAEL JACKSON

I've felt this way before, in my own heart. My body being pulled in directions I can't understand...

NANCY REAGAN

Michael, this is why we need you to lead the way. You're the only one who can hear the heart beating.

MICHAEL JACKSON

I'm beginning to understand why. I'll put the heart in my hands, but then what?

PRINCESS DIANA

Listen to me, no matter what, you are not to kill it.

NANCY REAGAN

You're to dip these Dior gowns into the blood in the MotherHeart's left ventricle.

PRINCESS DIANA

Without waking it.

NANCY REAGAN

Then you and Bubbles will put your mouths around two pulsing arteries and blow.

PRINCESS DIANA

Or you may be able to sing. We're not exactly sure—

NANCY SINATRA

Stop right there, Nancy Reagan and Princess Diana.

> *NANCY SINATRA holds two deadly boots in her hand, pointing directly at the women's hearts and also Michael Jackson's. BUBBLES rushes to Michael's middle, crashing him onto the floor and out of deadly range as if he were a Secret Service agent saving a president who used to star in Westerns.*

PRINCESS DIANA

Nancy! Do something!

NANCY SINATRA

I know exactly what you're up to, and I'll do anything to stop you, Awful Nancy.

NANCY REAGAN

Dive, Michael. Now!

> *MICHAEL JACKSON, BUBBLES, and RONALD REAGAN hold hands and jump into the ocean feet first. Splash!*

NANCY SINATRA

Oh god, where are they going?

PRINCESS DIANA

To the MotherHeart!

NANCY SINATRA

Nancy, you've got to stop them. They'll be trapped there forever!

NANCY REAGAN

This isn't your story to tell, other Nancy.

NANCY SINATRA

To think my Daddy loved you.

NANCY REAGAN

Take care, stupid girl! You are simply another version of me.

NANCY SINATRA

You are me.../

PRINCESS DIANA/NANCY REAGAN

What? / YES.

NANCY REAGAN

All of you, *shut up*. I need silence to think for all three of us at once.
Your existence depends on my denial.

PRINCESS DIANA

Nancy, don't hurt us— Please—

> *NANCY REAGAN, NANCY SINATRA, and PRINCESS DIANA*
> *wrestle one another in a violent tumble on the floor. Eventually they*
> *sync and spin somersaults through the infinite air, becoming One*
> *Woman Under God.*

NANCY SINATRA

We'll— We'll have to cover this up.

PRINCESS DIANA

What about Michael?

NANCY REAGAN

Yes, perfect. We'll blame him.

PRINCESS DIANA

But what if he comes back? He might come back...

NANCY SINATRA

Oh God, no, look... What *are* we?

PRINCESS DIANA

Now we're the same thing.

NANCY SINATRA

What will we do?

NANCY REAGAN

We'll become whatever we have to.

MOTHERS AND LOVERS

•

"Michael, you'll make an incredible mother one day,"

Diana would often babble, her beautiful hands busy with
a crucial but trivial task. Rinsing a dish, dusting a table.

The way she'd pull the curtains back
nearly stopped my clock every time.

FÉLIX GONZÁLEZ-TORRES JAN 9 1996

It is ironic then that for these two seminal decades
I was most intimate with Diana Ross and Nancy Reagan,

for the former is one of the greatest mothers and
the latter was notoriously, horribly messy.

["Alzheimer's brings people together." Cardboard.
Box Bin 11.]

Nancy and daughter Patti reconcile only after Ronald's official diagnosis with Alzheimer's
in 1994.

I often wished that I fell somewhere on the spectrum
halfway between them, but of course I wouldn't have

children until 1997, and even now, I'm hardly
anyone's mother in a conventional sense.

For most of my career the press
celebrated me as a boy-child,

my dancing an innovative jungle step
in the eyes of white critics.

FREDDIE MERCURY NOV 24 1991

One day Nancy went to theorizing that the figure Mowgli
was based on my early performances with my brothers.

I shook my head, desperate for her to
understand the timeline of our current era.

Eventually she conceded out of convenience:
"Alright, perhaps they were modeling after La Toya."

Apropos of her homespun prejudice,
Nancy's stories were always already

personal Yahtzees. She didn't ever
have to roll the dice.

[Personal materials. Paper.
File Folder Z-2.]

High-ranking officials illegally re-route Department of Housing and Urban Development
low-income housing grants to Reagan campaign contributors and Republican lobbyists.
The HUD grant rigging is not exposed until Reagan leaves office. Despite sixteen
convictions including James G. Watt's indictment on 24 felony counts, neither he nor
most of the fifteen other guilty parties spend time in jail.

Because it was shocking to outsiders how much
Janet resembled me, our mother always forced me

even at a young age to announce myself last.
This way, I resembled Janet, not the other way around.

Also just look at my lines.

WILLI SMITH APRIL 17 1987

There was a feeling in me like a mother.
I wanted to be decimated.

MARK MORRISROE JULY 24 1989

["Oliver North's Daddy Fantasies."
Zines, Box Bin 3.]

The night before Reagan's reelection, an Office of Public Diplomacy hoax circulates through the media that Soviet fighter jets have arrived in Nicaragua.

Ronald Reagan's arms conflicts, illegal invasions, secret wars, and support of counter-revolutionary death squads result in genocide, civil war, and brutality violating international law in Nicaragua, Guatemala, El Salvador, Grenada, Libya, Iraq, Iran, and Afghanistan.

Mass death (see also: *starvation*)
was to be ignored in those days—

the tail between the legs of two cities:
New York and D.C.

["Black Is Still Beautiful." Cardboard.
Box Bin C.]

In his 1976 campaign speech, Reagan evokes the new trope of the welfare queen to stoke hysteria about black women abusing the system. Over the course of his political career, Reagan opposes the Civil Rights Act of 1964, the Voting Rights Act of 1965, and the Fair Housing Act of 1968. He initially opposes the national holiday honoring Dr. Martin Luther King, Jr.

I rang Nancy that evening to say, "Darling,
I have had it. I'm relocating to Wonderland."

The old gin bottles hit salt water like a tea party,
a falling of the guard. Just before I settled the

receiver back into its holster,
a small specimen of my brain

thought I heard Nancy clarify,
with trepidation, "*Bahrain*?"

NANCY AT NOON

•

At the site of the lie, deep within her kingdom of infection, Nancy gazes down at the drowsy farmyard. She and her horse are heading westward across the swells at a swift pace. Come high noon, she will be independent, a mere particle of the universe.

She isn't too worried. Nancy can move between cells.

I've been sitting in my room for six years. For me, our meeting feels inevitable. I live for her arrival.

Nancy doesn't have to pray. She is certain her existence will not be disrupted. Life on the ranch will remain a tumble of cottonwood groves, rustling herds, ruins of the red rocks. A quick survey of the landscape establishes internal calm. She is doing this for her family: Ronnie and the kids.

Before all of this, I was, in my small scene, a beloved host. Dinner parties I arranged in cycles. Impromptu cocktails after the show became transcendent encounters under my hand. My secret?

Entertaining at home requires an imperceptible element of enchantment.

Some two hours later, a strange rider appears just short of the horizon. Nancy hopes he won't mix with her mission. She can finally see, up ahead, her destination of Dodge. The riders form together an arrow aimed at the town's purple haze.

The new American music celebrates the gold rush of white expansion. Some of Nancy's favorite composers are gays who feared revisionism. Aaron Copland and Virgil Thomson had divergent approaches to atonal music as well as homosexuality.

The sun polishes the alfalfa fields in a hazy gloss. As she nears the gates of the town, Nancy considers the mystery rider. She observes that the rider wears black leather—a misplaced samurai or a storm, smoking. Nancy reconsiders her thoughtful combination of denim trousers and matching collared shirt. Her beige gardening hat for shade. Tomorrow she'll take her red gingham on the town. For a moment, she is dreaming and she wonders whether or not they are alive.

"It must be coming on noon," Nancy tells herself, explaining away the heat, her delirium.

What felt like a joke is not anymore.

A photograph seems the animation of truth. The one protected in her busted satchel depicts an unknown man on a horse. He wears a pressed white shirt tucked into red slacks. He smiles up at the vast blue sky with arms outstretched. He looks like the future.

The day he died the sun burned solid gold.

My grief was fathomless. Strange beliefs redrew the boundary around my wild heart.

There are several images of Michael Jackson on a horse, including Kehinde Wiley's Napoleonic epic, *Equestrian Portrait of King Philip II (Michael Jackson)*. Jackson commissioned the piece but never lived to see it.

Shadows lengthen down the sage slope. Nancy figured for a storm on the edge of the horizon. Disaster seemed to hang everywhere, a queer custom ingrained in the weather.

Soon I began to hear things I wouldn't have heard otherwise. Things I had denied.

I make out a clear path to Dodge. I know who she is before she knows me. That denim-clad show cow taught me how to hide.

Nancy sees now that the rider was tracking her, matching her progress across the low plain almost exactly. There came to her the startling conviction that she must bond with the rider or find a more defensive pathway. Colder and tighter stretched the skin over her face.

At the end of *High Noon* (1952), Amy shoots Pierce from behind.

While he was writing the screenplay for *High Noon*, Carl Foreman was called before the House Un-American Activities Committee. He refused to give names to the committee, was blacklisted, and moved to England, where he pseudonymously co-wrote *The Bridge on the River Kwai* (1957) with another blacklisted Hollywood screenwriter, Michael Wilson. In 1984, they were honored posthumously for the Academy Award the screenplay received under other names.

The sun of this blazing western beats down on the midday dirt, and everything as far as the riders can see is near dying of thirst. Vision is the barrel of a rifle, scoping the storefronts of the town, careening along these rails of perspective.

Close to tipping off, Nancy's hoping for a train stop at that pinpoint on the horizon. She hopes to see it first. Its function is to hold the imagination and pull it farther west, through the suction tube of fantasy that goes from her mouth to his. Ronnie.

Nancy knows it does no good to invoke Biblical allusions. There won't be a martyr; Nancy won't be crucified. Even with a throat as dry as hers she can still whistle the opening bars of "Trust and Obey."

For the rider in leather, every pore feels like a tiny wound or window; the only places from which the plumes of thick black smoke can escape, the fire raging just beneath the parched skin covering arms, neck, broken face.

Both ride along nodding through exhaustion. They are awakened once the sun pours a golden stream of light through the great stone arch. The horses halt, nostrils flaring.

The riders tumble from their horses like sacks of feed, then shuffle around the beasts to square off. Nancy's white, glistening eyes meet the rider's dark slit for seeing. She reaches out toward it when suddenly, as she inspects the rider more closely, something checks her, and as quickly all her joy flees, with it her color, the memories and myths.

The rider takes a dozen paces and turns back to face
Nancy.

By degrees she is waning.

I return to an original thought, that my brains might be exposed to the sun, a can of beans cooking in the top of my head.

A short spasm rocks through me. I let my head fall back until my neck burns. Then, I do it.

I look directly into the sun with my hand on an empty holster.

In a flash there are five thousand Nancies replicating in my eyes, my brain. My stomach turns and dumps itself out. An entire species of acquired charms invades my space; Nancy induces hallucination at the viral spike. She's blazing through my borders. Faced with the assembly of her life, she is forced to release.

The rider's head is a gold rush of sunlight. Nancy shades her eyes with a trembling hand, breathing the dust of the border town in through her nose, the pungent stab of glue.

Dodge isn't a real place. The settler fantasy main street for a western colossus is the cover of the *High Noon* DVD. In her camouflage, Nancy is quickly shrinking.

She continues to shrink until she's only visible between the rider's legs.

The rider is wearing chaps.

The rider is standing in a gay bar in San Francisco in 1988.

"Smooth Criminal" is on the radio.

Down in her canyon of obliviousness, Nancy is so small that she can only see my silhouette. It takes her several minutes, but she finally recognizes me.

Her face puffs crimson. She turns in an instant.

Don't leave me, Nancy begs. I need you to survive.

There's nothing left for you to feed on, I try to say

inside the mirror

nothing comes out

a sparkling disco ball

strands of fake hair in the dust

FOOTSTEPS IN THE DARK

•

I was pissed at Nancy and Ronald.
I walked the moonlit trail for an hour

trying to shake their racist garbage
out of my pant leg. I dreamed at night that

those two were the bugs planted all around my house.
I decided I would never talk to them again, as I was
dialing

Nancy's number, which was incredibly long—
filled with pass codes and god knows what.

It occurred to me as I pushed the keys
that some of the numbers were probably me,

digits alerting them that Michael Jackson was calling.

CLÁUDIA WONDER NOV 26 2010

It rang and rang.

Finally, I heard a live breath
on the end of the line.

I waited.

MARTIN WONG AUG 12 1999

I whispered, "Nancy? It's Michael."

ALVIN AILEY DEC 1 1989

Breath again. I could be sure
the call had gone through,

the line was live.

ESQUERITA OCT 23 1986

"Nancy, it's me,
Michael. May I

speak with Nancy,
Nancy Reagan?"

CHLOE DZUBILO FEB 18 2011

The noise I heard next

reminded me of textbooks

MICHEL FOUCAULT JUNE 25 1984

electrified screams

and then

ANTÓNIO VARIAÇÕES JUNE 13 1984

the illustration of

Benjamin Franklin

SAM WAGSTAFF JAN 14 1987

147

discovering electricity

JACK SMITH SEP 25 1989

with a kite

PATRICK KELLY JAN 1 1990

.

I was afraid, excited.

ED MOCK APRIL 25 1986

This is what it's like
to have a friend.

IRIS DE LA CRUZ MAY 11 1990

"Nancy, this is Michael.
Your friend—Nancy—Michael.

LOU SULLIVAN MARCH 2 1991

Nancy is,
this is

Nancy."

REZA ABDOH MAY 12 1995

In an instant, I dropped the phone, which had become

scorching hot, a live flame that burnt the carpet

in the shape of a telephone receiver.

In the background of my eye, I fantasized

Nancy's head backlit by a blazing fire.

She was a *Poltergeist* (1982), a vision received.

MICHAEL JACKSON'S
THRILLER

•

Week I

you	try
to	scream

Nothing can   keep me

keep me from you

Week 9

To make more meaning

reveal all arrangements

as underbellies

the graveyard wish

of grief

to come out of ground

my short-sightedness

skin push away skin

the evil lurking in the dark

Week 15

The negative space on my first album cover was one key

A tiger tore at my sense of origin before I turned 24

And here we are, already at the number

$2 per album

                           make of me my royalties and grill

                           the half moon, your night smile

                           parade

                           stomps my trapped face a surprise

                           in and ever I'm synchronized

Home

worm

Lyricism inverts—my own and the world's desires

Their hunch: thinking they were looking for me

a boy not normal enough, easily buried to aliens

They made a science fiction mistaking helmet

seeing easy where my elegance repelled

I was boring through the sides

of their monuments

with my weirdness

Week 24

A casket   the mask of the first hibernation

A musket

A man   I harnessed a glamour I no longer desired

even if as a woman I wanted to take the problem in how had I become
so princely

through the fashionable obscuring of my face they had constructed for
me a me

To everyone's surprise I was beautiful

falsetto   bestseller

no wind   no rain

use my tunnel as a light   up on the racks with

for talent to move through   black crows where nothing

me baby I want to   hurts but sunbeam and gin

I lose   my moves

                    how to get loose

With meditation taking up more and more of my time
I noticed in Week 27

I was against something, or within it

Meditation notes from week 28-32
consist mostly of signs although
occasionally words creep vine-like
across the page. My fingers warm
over those that fit merely one letter

I read by making sense over the light
of twenty pages: one word, *laborious*,
what with the euphoria of rotation

Weeks 32 and 33
when the black hole
hushed all around me

I slipped into it like a cat suit
without constraint, without judgment

Week 35

The costume had become my body

I moved through the world either girl or ghoul but seriously

Not Death but definitely Close

Making a face beneath my other face

sealing it with one precious lick of lip

I spit

                                                            I wail

                                                    under the moonlight

inside the war of the boy body the world's
violence is compressed within eggshell I told
La Toya I could hold the egg without breaking it
but I got an odd one you have to be careful not to
get one that's already cracked I know some eggs
have blood inside and that's okay mother says
never throw out an egg this boy's body these faces
that never open their smiles the egg holds itself
closed with spiral bands of tissue I was always
very delicate inside the yolk is suspended the
mix-up of adult and child such clever membrane
so tenuous in the balance you can eat it

there's a wide variation although at first I think
they are all the same the excitement is never knowing
what I'm getting although I can rely on the fact that
the punishment is coming she says imagine you're
the egg being beaten imagine you're the egg being
beaten use your imagination the muscled membrane
hard-boiled as an egg a wet soggy goop that makes a
mess and then there are the ones in between the shell and
the yolk baby and adult something very white whiter than
marshmallow no fat all protein and it feeds me I feed on it

Week 36

I see no one and feel no one
I float over all things as nothing, a wish

Without grace

I accumulate

a stormy test tube

Week 37

I said I'm not like other guys

Me little wizard zombie

Legs like a penis spin to get down

You can, you can't in chorus

Watch I want to win child

I want you to give in

Here I begin out in the field — the old scarecrow —

A bimbo with bad news

Bringing me the blues

Not with the whip again the star encrusted

The yellow road in occult out of gas

I like you 10 MPH

Scratches rings on your fingers

I hope you like scripts girl

Who's captive   Who's the boss

              legendary creature

        attired in candy technicolor

              bring me the moon

    the cat eyes   the claws

                fighting to survive inside a killer
You're fighting to survive   a killer
You're fighting to survive inside a killer
You're   to survive inside a killer
You're fighting to survive inside a killer
You're fighting to survive inside a killer
You're fighting to survive inside a killer
You're fighting to   inside a killer
You're fighting to survive inside a killer
You're fighting to survive inside a killer
You're fighting to survive inside a killer
You're fighting to survive inside   killer
You're fighting to survive inside a killer
You're fighting   survive inside a killer
You're fighting to survive inside

NANCY AT BULGARI

•

On the cusp of a hoax Nancy wavers.

Should she choose the opal brooch

or the pearl and diamond ear clips?

What year is it?

Did Nancy arrive from Washington?

From Sacramento?

Ask anyone, anywhere, and they'll tell you.

After the glory years, all of these people

became mere shadows of themselves.

But not Nancy.

Nancy is everywhere.

She is not over.

ACKNOWLEDGMENTS

•

Deep gratitude to the team at Futurepoem, especially Dan Machlin and the 2017 guest editors Monica McClure, Pierre Joris, and Claudia La Rocco. Admiration and forever thanks to my fabulous editor Carly Dashiell, who tended to my obsessions with great insight, elegance, and care. Miguel Gutierrez, Robert Glück, Claudia La Rocco, and Samuel R. Delany, love and thanks for your generosity and support.

This book began as a series of hauntings that I got to process within the community of 2014 Poets House fellows. Special thanks to Lara Lorenzo, Aeliana Nicole, Wo Chan, and Vincent Toro; to J. Mae Barizo who asked me, a year later, whatever happened to my Nancy poems.

Over the years, I've received feedback on this manuscript from brilliant friends: Mónica de la Torre, Aldrin Valdez, Emmett Ramstad, Jason Zuzga, Timothy Liu, Selby W. Schwartz, Tisa Bryant, and Robert Glück. Tremendous thanks to Saretta Morgan and Ari Banias who came through as readers of the final manuscript.

Thank you to my mentors: Sarah Schulman, David Halperin, Esther Newton, and Holly Hughes. For sons and lovers, Stephen Ira and Kevin Killian. Thank you to my students, for every revelation.

At last, endless love to the queen Diana Cage, who makes everything possible.

This is for you.

NOTES

•

RED RIBBON

A GALLERY
maxecrandall.com/work/nancy-reagans/

I find my epigraphs in David Román's *Acts of Intervention: Performance, Gay Culture, and AIDS* (Indiana UP, 1998) and an interview with Kimberlé W. Crenshaw by Sheila Thomas titled "Intersectionality: The Double Bind of Race and Gender," published in *Perspectives* (2004).

DAZED, FROM WHICH DISTRACTION

mouth of the Hudson...
Bob Hope at the July 4, 1986 rededication of the Statue of Liberty. "AIDS in New York: A Biography." *New York Magazine*, online.

Isn't it funny...
Nancy Reagan. *I Love You Ronnie: The Letters of Ronald Reagan to Nancy Reagan.* Random House, 2000.

ALL WAYS, A HUNTED

Fake fire alarm at the governor's mansion...
"Remembering Carmichael's 'Taj Mahal' Exec Mansion." *Valcom News*, online.

the Rose Garden ceremony...
Tricia's Wedding (film), 1971.

The gold chains are a symbol...
Mr. T. *Mr T: The Man with the Gold: An Autobiography.* St. Martins Press, 1984.

raided premises...
Historic sign hanging inside the door to the Stonewall Inn. See Jake Offenhartz, "Police Commissioner Apologizes for NYPD Raid of Stonewall." *Gothamist*, online.

JANET SPEAKS

This chapter is partially composed, reworked, and remixed from Susan Elsa's website archangelmichael777.wordpress.com, found text located as a guide on how to become someone else inside oneself. "We come into array."—Susan Elsa

If I die forget burial...
David Wojnarowicz's black leather jacket

MY OWN PRIVATE PARADOX

Rock Hudson had AIDS and was trying to reach her...
See Chris Geidner's *Buzzfeed* article, "Nancy Reagan Turned Down Rock Hudson's Plea For Help Nine Weeks Before He Died."

It is counterproductive...
United States National Archives and Records Administration Federal Register Office. *Weekly Compilation of Presidential Documents*, Volume 20, Issues 40-52. Page 1881.

She came at me in sections...
Arthur Schwartz and Howard Dietz. "Girl Hunt Ballet" in *The Band Wagon* (film), 1953. Michael Jackson included these lyrics in his 1991 song "Dangerous."

IRRESISTIBLE FORCES

"Nicaragua Must Survive"
Archival entry for poster made by Luisa Amanda Espinoza and Orlando Valenzuela circa 1985. Center for the Study of Political Graphics, online.

I was going to ask if this interview...
Margaret Randall. *When I Look into the Mirror and See You: Women, Terror, and Resistance.* Rutgers University Press, 2002.

African Americans are incarcerated in state prisons...
Ashley Nellis. "The Color of Justice: Racial and Ethnic Disparity in State Prisons." The Sentencing Project, 2016. Available online.

Dora Maria the warrior girl who blasted the tyrant's heart...
Margaret Randall. *Sandino's Daughters.* New Star Books, 1981.

The development of colonial cities...
See Sousa JDd, Müller V, Lemey P, Vandamme A-M. "High GUD Incidence in the Early 20th Century Created a Particularly Permissive Time Window for the Origin and Initial Spread of Epidemic HIV Strains." *PLOS ONE* 5.4 (2010).

JUST SAY AIDS

Reagan intimate William F. Buckley...
See William F. Buckley, Jr. "Crucial Steps in Combating the Aids Epidemic; Identify All the Carriers." *The New York Times*, March 18, 1986.

technically limb-like...
See Paul Thek. *Warrior's Leg*, 1966-67. From the series *Technological Reliquaries*.

as if my tail were a thousand...
See Steve Abbott. *The Lizard Club*. Autonomedia, 1993. Thanks to Brenda Iijima.

They don't know how it is with us...
Nancy Reagan with William Novak. *My Turn: The Memoirs of Nancy Reagan*. Random House, 1989.

SWORN TO SECRECY

White House recipe card.
Courtesy of Jason Zuzga.

The lone photograph...
See Joan Quigley. *"What Does Joan Say?" My Seven Years as White House Astrologer to Nancy and Ronald Reagan*. Birch Lane Press, 1990.

but the aura itself...
See Walter Benjamin, "The Work of Art in the Age of Mechanical Reproduction." *Illuminations*. Schocken Books, 1968.

NANCY AT NOON

This chapter repurposes text from Zane Grey's *Riders of the Purple Sage* (1912).

AMERICA'S BRAIN

A FILM FESTIVAL

2007: Nelson George's *Life Support*

1953: Felix E. Feist's *Donovan's Brain*

2012: Jim Hubbard and Sarah Schulman's *United in Anger: A History of ACT UP*

1999: Pedro Almodóvar's *All About My Mother*

1984: "Michael Jackson's hair caught fire" on *YouTube*

1958: Fred F. Sears's *Crash Landing*

2018: Dan Krauss's *5B*

1992: Marlon Riggs's *Non, Je Ne Regrette Rien (No Regret)*

1940: March of Dimes fundraiser short *The Crippler* [sic]

1987: Alexandra Juhasz with Jean Carlomusto *Living with AIDS: Women and AIDS*. Available online.

Ongoing: Visual AIDS's *Day With(out) Art* video commissions

MICHAEL JACKSON'S *THRILLER*

This chapter features lyrics from Michael Jackson's "Thriller" and Diana Ross's "Ain't No Mountain High Enough" and builds from images in *The Wiz* (1978).

SELECTED SOURCES

•

Abdoh, Reza, director. *Bogeyman*. dar a luz productions, videographer
Adam Soch, Los Angeles Theater Center, August 29, 1991.
https:// vimeo.com/156807754

Ahmed, Sara. "Queer Feelings." *The Cultural Politics of Emotions*. Routledge,
2004. 144-167.

Beam, Joseph (ed). *In the Life: A Black Gay Anthology*. Second Edition.
Redbone Press, 2007. [1986]

Bellamy, Dodie. *The Letters of Mina Harker*. Hard Press, 1998.

Beneš, Barton Lidicé. *Art Museum*, 1992-1999. Wood, paper, ink,
plexiglass.

Brother(hood) Dance!, Orlando Zane Hunter and Ricarrdo Valentine.
how to survive a plague. St. Marks Church, New York, November 17-
19, 2016.

Coan, Jamie Shearn, Ishmael Houston-Jones, and Will Rawls, editors.
Lost and Found: Dance, New York, HIV/AIDS, Then and Now. Danspace
Project Platform, 2016.

Cohen, Cathy J. *The Boundaries of Blackness: AIDS and the Breakdown of Black
Politics*. University of Chicago Press, 1999.

Crenshaw, Kimberlé. Interview with Sheila Thomas.
"Intersectionality: The Double Bind of Race and Gender,"
Perspectives 12.4, 2004.

Crimp, Douglas with Adam Rolston. *AIDS Demographics*. Bay Press, 1990.

Delany, Samuel R. *Dahlgren*. Knopf Doubleday Publishing Group,
2001. [1974]

Finkelstein, Avram. *After Silence: A History of AIDS through Its Images*.
University of California Press, 2018.

Fleetwood, Nicole R. *On Racial Icons: Blackness and the Public Imagination*. Rutgers University Press, 2015.

Glück, Robert. *Margery Kempe*. High Risk Books, 1994.

Gutierrez, Miguel and Ishmael Houston-Jones. *Variations on Themes from Lost and Found: Scenes from a Life and other works by John Bernd*. St. Marks Church, New York, November 3-5, 2016.

Halperin, David. *How to Be Gay*. The Belknap Press of Harvard University Press, 2012.

Jolivette, Andrew J. *Indian Blood: HIV and Colonial Trauma in San Francisco's Two-Spirit Community*. University of Washington Press, 2016.

Juhasz, Alexandra. *AIDS TV: Identity, Community, and Alternative Video*. Duke University Press, 1995.

Kerr, Theodore (Ted). "AIDS 1969: HIV, History, and Race." *Drain Magazine*, http://drainmag.com/aids-1969-hiv-history-and-race/.

Leonard, Zoe. *Strange Fruit (for David)*. 1992-1997. 295 banana, orange, grapefruit, lemon, and avocado peels, thread, zippers, buttons, sinew, needles, plastic, wire, stickers, fabric, trim, wax.

Lemebel, Pedro. *My Tender Matador*. Translated by Katherine Silver. Grove Press, 2003. [1985]

Long, Charles Ryan. *Nancy Reagan Is Killing Me*. The Center for Book, Paper & Print Columbia College Chicago, 2016.

McCruer, Robert. "Crip." *Keywords for Radicals*: The Contested Vocabulary of Late-Capitalist Struggle (eds Kelly Fritsch, Clare O'Connor, and AK Thomson). AK Press, 2016.

McKay, Richard A. *Patient Zero and the Making of the AIDS Epidemic*. The University of Chicago Press, 2017.

Nomi, Klaus. *Za Bakdaz: The Unfinished Opera*. Heliocentric, 2006.

Patton, Cindy. *Globalizing AIDS*. University of Minnesota Press, 2002.

Román, David. *Acts of Intervention: Performance, Gay Culture, and AIDS*. Indiana University Press, 1998.

Schulman, Sarah. *The Gentrification of the Mind: Witness to a Lost Generation*. University of California Press, 2013.

Schwartz, Selby W. *The Bodies of Others: Drag Dance and its Afterlives*. University of Michigan Press, 2019.

Sherlock, Alexandra. "Larger Than Life: Digital Resurrection and the Re-Enchantment of Society." *The Information Society* 29.3 (2013): 164-176.

Woubshet, Dagmawi. *The Calendar of Loss: Race, Sexuality, and Mourning in the Early Era of AIDS*. Johns Hopkins University Press, 2015.

RESOURCES

•

ACT UP Oral History Project / actuporalhistory.org

@theaidsmemorial

Center for the Study of Political Graphics / politicalgraphics.org

The Freedom Archives / freedomarchives.org

A Gender Variance Who's Who / zagria.blogspot.com

POZ / poz.com

Sentencing Project / sentencingproject.org

Sero Project / seroproject.com

Visual AIDS / visualaids.org

What Would an HIV Doula Do? / hivdoula.work/

This first edition, first printing, includes 26 limited edition copies signed by the author and lettered a-z.